LUPUS DISEASE

LIVING WELL WITH LUPUS

DR HARRY U SCHAEFER

COPYRIGHT

DEDICATION

Lupus patients' resiliency demonstrates the strength of the human spirit. This book is dedicated to you, and I hope it brings you understanding, optimism, and the strength to thrive in the face of obstacles.

PREFACE

As a physician specializing in autoimmune diseases, I have seen firsthand the profound impact that lupus can have on the lives of those it touches. This complex, unpredictable condition challenges not only the individuals diagnosed with it, but also their families, friends, and healthcare teams. Lupus is a disease that does not follow a straightforward path, and its symptoms vary widely, making each case as unique as the person living with it.

This book is a reflection of my years of working with lupus patients, combined with the latest medical knowledge about the disease. It is my goal to offer insight into the medical, emotional, and practical aspects of living with lupus, not just as a condition to be treated, but as a part of everyday life that requires understanding, patience, and resilience. My approach in writing this book was guided by one simple principle: to empower individuals living with lupus to better understand their condition and to provide them with the tools to actively participate in their care.

Lupus is often misunderstood, even within the medical community. Its symptoms mimic those of many other diseases, and its invisible nature can make it difficult for others to grasp the full extent of what someone with lupus experiences. With this book, I hope to demystify the disease, provide clarity, and offer practical strategies for managing it effectively.

This journey through lupus is not just about coping; it's about thriving despite the challenges. Whether you are someone newly diagnosed, a long-time lupus warrior, or a caregiver or healthcare professional seeking to better understand the disease, this book is written with you in mind. It covers a range of topics symptom management, navigating flare-ups, emotional well-being, and long-term care each designed to help individuals find a path forward that works for them.

Ultimately, this book is about hope. Lupus, while life-altering, does not define a person's future. With advances in medicine and a deeper understanding of the disease, individuals living with lupus today have more options and resources than ever before. My hope is that this book will serve as a guide, offering not just medical advice, but encouragement and support as you navigate your unique journey with lupus.

Dr. Harry U. Schaefer
Physician Specialist

AUTHOR BIOGEOGRAPHY

Dr Harry U. Schaefer is a distinguished author and physician, recognized for his extensive work in the field of autoimmune diseases and chronic illness management. With a passion for simplifying complex medical conditions, Schaefer has written several acclaimed books, making vital health information accessible to readers worldwide. His writings empower individuals with chronic conditions, helping them navigate their diagnoses with confidence and clarity.

Schaefer's academic journey began at University of California, San Francisco, where he earned his medical degree, specializing in internal medicine and autoimmune disorders. He further honed his expertise with advanced training and research, making significant contributions to the understanding of lupus and other related conditions. Throughout his career, he has remained dedicated to patient education, believing that informed patients make the best decisions for their health.

Beyond his medical career, Schaefer is a devoted family man. Balancing his professional achievements with his personal life, he draws inspiration from his family's unwavering support, which fuels his commitment to helping others. His approach to both life and medicine is driven by a desire to provide practical, compassionate solutions to the challenges that chronic illness presents.

Schaefer's books have resonated with readers on Amazon for their clarity, thoroughness, and practical insights. He believes that while medical expertise is crucial, the human element understanding the emotional and physical impact of illness is just as important. His works are more than guides; they are companions for anyone navigating the complexities of chronic disease.

Whether you're a patient, caregiver, or medical professional, Dr Harry U. Schaefer's books offer valuable knowledge and hope, making him a trusted voice in health and wellness literature.

Table of contents

THERE'S ALWAYS HOPE

For a start I would love to share with you the story of Jessica, a young Lady who has been thriving even with a diagnosed Lupus. During my research with my Team we found out how encouraging her story would be if shared.

Her story showcases hope and motivation Which highlights resilience and reminds others that they are not defined by their illness.Hearing or reading this Story fosters a sense of community, reduces feelings of isolation, and provides practical coping tools.

At 28, Jessica Williams had become an expert in managing her life with lupus, a condition diagnosed three years earlier that had initially shaken her world. Once a vibrant girl working as a graphic designer during a bustling city, she faced challenges that tested her resilience. Yet, through determination and self-discovery, Jessica not only learned to live with lupus but also to thrive despite it.

In the beginning, the diagnosis felt kind of a dark cloud hovering over her. The constant fatigue, joint pain, and unpredictable flares disrupted her daily routine and left her feeling isolated. Friends and colleagues struggled to understand her invisible illness, often making casual comments that stung. "You don't look sick," they could say, leaving her to desire she was constantly defending her reality.

Determined to not let lupus define her, Jessica sought knowledge. She immersed herself in research, reading articles and joining online forums where others shared their experiences. It was here that she discovered a community of people who understood her struggles, and slowly, she began to feel less alone. Encouraged by their stories, Jessica sought out a rheumatologist who specialized in autoimmune diseases. Together, they developed a treatment plan that included medication, regular exercise, and a spotlight on nutrition.

With her new routine, Jessica embraced a healthier lifestyle. She started cooking wholesome meals, learning to balance her love for food with anti-inflammatory ingredients. It had been a revelation to urge how foods like leafy greens, nuts, and fatty fish could boost her energy levels and help manage her symptoms. Cooking became therapeutic, transforming her kitchen into a neighborhood of creativity and nourishment.

She as well joined a neighborhood yoga studio, drawn to the gentle movements and specialize in mindfulness. Although the first few classes were challenging, she quickly noticed the benefits. Yoga not only helped alongside her physical symptoms but also provided a mental escape, allowing her to center herself during difficult days. As she became more attuned to her body, she learned to acknowledge the signs of an impending flare, adjusting her activities accordingly.

Socially, Jessica found her voice. She began to share her experiences openly with friends and family, educating them about lupus and thus the impact it had on her life. To her surprise, their support grew stronger.

Friends started accompanying her to yoga classes, and family gatherings transformed into moments of understanding rather than awkwardness. Her vulnerability sparked meaningful conversations, helping others to know the unseen battles people face.

With newfound confidence, Jessica took a leap of faith and launched her own freelance graphic design business. She envisioned a flexible career that allowed her to work from home on days when fatigue set in. The transition wasn't without its hurdles, but her passion for design fueled her perseverance. Each completed project was a testament to her resilience and skill to thrive despite her health challenges.

As her business flourished, she also became an advocate for lupus awareness. She shared her story on social media, participated in local events, and contributed to online discussions, going to shed light on the realities of living with an invisible illness. Her openness resonated with many, and she or he or he found purpose in helping others navigate their journeys.

Today, Jessica stands as a logo of strength and hope. She embraces life with lupus, armed with knowledge, community, and an unwavering spirit. Through her challenges, she has learned that thriving isn't merely about overcoming obstacles but about redefining what it means to live fully, authentically, and unapologetically.

I bet you'll find this 'quick read' useful for you and anyone living with Lupus.

Happy study.

INTRODUCTION

UNDERSTANDING LUPUS DISEASE IN THE UNITED STATES

Let's begin this journey looking at some statistics. Lupus is a chronic autoimmune disorder, Which affects an estimated 1.5 million people within the US alone.

Although it's a worldwide health issue, its impact on Americans, particularly women and minorities, presents a singular set of challenges. Despite its prevalence, lupus remains a condition that's widely misunderstood by the general public.

The disease, marked by its unpredictability and wide selection of symptoms, are often debilitating for those affected, often disrupting lifestyle in significant ways. This book is meant to offer readers a radical understanding of lupus, covering everything from its causes and symptoms to treatment options and therefore the personal experiences of those living with the disease.

The term "lupus" refers to several related diseases, the foremost common being systemic LE (SLE). Lupus occurs when the body's system, which normally defends against harmful invaders like bacteria and viruses, mistakenly attacks its own tissues. This internal confusion can cause widespread inflammation and damage to vital organs, including the guts, kidneys, skin, and brain. What makes lupus particularly difficult is its complexity: no two cases are exactly alike. Some patients may experience mild symptoms, while others face life-threatening complications. This variation often leaves patients, their families, and even healthcare providers struggling to know the complete scope of the disease.

What makes lupus tougher to manage within the US is the difficulty of diagnosing it early. Many of its symptoms, like fatigue, joint pain, and skin rashes, overlap with other common ailments. Due to this, it can take years for somebody with lupus to receive a correct diagnosis. This delay often results in unnecessary suffering and missed opportunities to start treatment, which may slow the disease's progression.

Lupus features a particular demographic pattern within the U.S., disproportionately affecting women, especially women of color. Around 90% of lupus patients are women, and African American, Hispanic, Asian, and Native American women are two to 3 times more likely to develop the disease than Caucasian women. The explanations behind this demographic disparity are still not fully understood. Researchers believe that genetics, environmental factors, and hormonal influences play a task, but much remains to be uncovered. This inequality in who gets lupus also raises critical questions on healthcare

access, as minorities often face additional barriers to receiving timely diagnoses and coverings.

Despite its serious nature, lupus isn't a widely discussed condition. Many of us outside of the medical field are unacquainted with its effects, which may make it difficult for patients to elucidate their illness or find the support they have. Unlike diseases like cancer or diabetes, lupus lacks an equivalent level of public awareness, and as a result, fewer resources are dedicated to lupus research and treatment development. This gap in understanding and funding has slowed progress in finding a cure or maybe simpler treatments.

Living with lupus is often isolating, particularly when symptoms are "invisible" to others. People with lupus often face skepticism or misunderstanding about their condition, especially during times of remission when symptoms could also be less noticeable. Flare-ups, however, can happen all of sudden, leaving patients exhausted or in pain with little outward sign of illness. This unpredictability can disrupt work, relationships, and daily routines, making it difficult for patients to plan their lives.

Managing lupus involves quite just treating physical symptoms. Because lupus may be a lifelong condition, those diagnosed with it must make long-term adjustments to their lifestyle. This will include learning to deal with chronic pain and fatigue, adhering to complex medication regimens, and making difficult choices about work, family life, and social activities. The emotional toll of lupus is

critical, with many patients facing anxiety, depression, and feelings of isolation. Access to psychological state resources is crucial, but many patients find it hard to seek out specialists who understand the unique psychological burdens of chronic illness.

Despite the challenges of lupus, progress is being made in understanding and treating the disease. In recent years, researchers have made important strides in identifying the underlying causes of lupus and developing new treatments that focus on specific aspects of the system. The introduction of biologic drugs, which help regulate the immune reaction, has provided hope for several lupus patients, offering an alternative to traditional treatments like corticosteroids, which accompany significant side effects. Still, the journey toward a cure is way from over, and more research is required to completely unlock the mysteries of this complex disease.

The lupus community within the US is growing stronger annually, with more patients, advocates, and researchers working together to boost awareness and push for better treatments. Advocacy organizations just like the Lupus Foundation of America have played a pivotal role in giving lupus patients a voice, promoting education, and securing funding for research. These efforts have already made a difference, with increased public awareness and government support for lupus-related healthcare initiatives. However, much work remains to be done. For patients living with lupus, every day may be a new challenge, but the continued efforts to know and combat the disease offer

hope for a brighter future.

This book aims to supply a comprehensive overview of lupus, particularly within the context of its impact on Americans. Each chapter will delve into a special aspect of the disease, from its biological mechanisms to the lived experiences of these who battle it daily. We'll explore the medical challenges of diagnosing and treating lupus, also because of the social, emotional, and financial burdens it places on patients and their families. Along the way, we'll also highlight the stories of people who have turned their personal battles with lupus into a source of strength, advocating for better healthcare and more research into this often-overlooked disease.

Whether you're someone living with lupus, a caregiver, a medical professional, or just someone curious about learning more about this complex disease, this book will provide you with valuable insights into lupus within the us. The goal is to teach, inform, and, above all, support those suffering from lupus by offering a clearer understanding of what they face and the way they will better manage their condition. Lupus could also be a chronic illness, but with better knowledge and stronger advocacy, we will improve the lives of those living with it and move closer to finding a cure.

CHAPTER 1

WHAT EXACTLY IS LUPUS?

Lupus as we started earlier is a chronic autoimmune disorder that affects many people worldwide, with a big number residing within the US. At its core, lupus occurs when the body's system, which usually protects against infections and diseases, mistakenly attacks healthy tissues and organs. This autoimmune response results in inflammation, pain, and damage to varied parts of the body, including the joints, skin, kidneys, heart, lungs, and brain. While lupus manifests differently in everyone, it often brings a mixture of challenging symptoms which will significantly disrupt lifestyle.

The Role of the system in Lupus

To understand lupus, it's essential to first grasp the immune system's normal function. During a healthy person, the system acts because of the body's defense reaction. It produces proteins called antibodies, which recognize and neutralize foreign invaders like bacteria and viruses. These antibodies are a part of a posh system that identifies and destroys harmful substances, while leaving healthy cells alone.

In people with lupus, this technique malfunctions. For reasons that aren't fully understood, the system becomes hyperactive and produces autoantibodies, which are antibodies that mistakenly attack the body's own tissues. The body treats its own cells and tissues as if they were invaders, resulting in inflammation and tissue damage. This immune confusion is what defines lupus and sets it aside from many other diseases. While other autoimmune diseases may target specific organs (such as the pancreas in type 1 diabetes or the thyroid in Hashimoto's thyroiditis), lupus is systemic. This suggests it can affect multiple organs and systems, making the disease unpredictable and difficult to manage.

TYPES OF LUPUS

There are several sorts of lupus, each with unique characteristics and implications for those affected. The foremost common form, systemic LE (SLE), is the one most frequently mentioned when people speak of lupus. However, there are other types, including cutaneous lupus, drug-induced lupus, and neonatal lupus.

Systemic LE (SLE):

SLE is the most prevalent and high sort of lupus, affecting multiple systems throughout the body. The hallmark of SLE is its unpredictable nature: patients experience "flare-ups" when symptoms worsen, followed by periods of remission when symptoms subside. The severity of SLE varies from person to person, with some individuals experiencing mild symptoms, while others face life-threatening complications. SLE can affect the skin, joints, kidneys, heart, lungs, brain, and blood vessels, making it a posh disease to diagnose and treat.

Cutaneous Lupus:

This form of lupus primarily affects the skin. The foremost recognizable symptom of cutaneous lupus may be a rash, which frequently appears on areas of the body exposed to sunlight. There are different subtypes of cutaneous lupus, with discoid lupus being one among the foremost common. Discoid lupus causes round, raised lesions which will leave scars, and although it primarily affects the skin, some people with discoid lupus may continue to develop SLE.

Another subtype, subacute cutaneous LE, causes red, scaly patches that always don't leave scars but are often quite uncomfortable.

Drug-Induced Lupus:

Some medications can trigger lupus-like symptoms in certain individuals. This condition is understood as drug-induced lupus. Unlike SLE, drug-induced lupus is typically temporary, and symptoms typically resolve once the offending medication is stopped. Common drugs related to this condition include certain vital sign medications, anti-seizure drugs, and antibiotics. The symptoms of drug-induced lupus are almost like those of SLE, but they're generally milder and less likely to cause long-term damage to organs.

Neonatal Lupus:

Though rare, neonatal lupus can occur when autoantibodies from a mother with lupus cross the placenta and affect the developing fetus. Infants with neonatal lupus may experience a rash, liver problems, or low blood corpuscle counts. In most cases, the symptoms disappear after a couple of months, and therefore the baby doesn't continue to develop lupus later in life. However, in rare cases, babies with neonatal lupus may have a heart disease called congenital Adams-Stokes syndrome, which may be life-threatening.

Symptoms of Lupus

Lupus is often referred to as "the great imitator" because its symptoms can resemble those of other diseases, like atrophic arthritis, fibromyalgia, and MS. The variability of symptoms, combined with their often subtle onset, makes lupus difficult to diagnose. Symptoms may appear suddenly or develop gradually over time. they will be mild or severe, and their intensity may fluctuate over time. Below are a number of the foremost common symptoms of lupus.

Fatigue:
One of the foremost prevalent symptoms, fatigue, are often overwhelming for those with lupus. It's not equivalent to simply feeling tired after an extended day; lupus-related fatigue is persistent and may significantly impact an individual's ability to function.

Joint Pain and Swelling:
Lupus frequently affects the joints, causing pain, stiffness, and swelling. These symptoms are often most noticeable within the morning or after periods of rest. Unlike atrophic arthritis, lupus-related joint pain tends to be less destructive to the joints, although it can still be debilitating.

Skin Rashes:
Skin issues are common in lupus, particularly a butterfly-shaped rash that spreads across the cheeks and nose. This characteristic rash, referred to as a malar rash, often appears or worsens after sun exposure.

Other sorts of rashes can also occur, particularly on areas of the body exposed to sunlight.

Kidney Problems:
Lupus nephritis, or inflammation of the kidneys, may be a serious complication that affects up to 60% of individuals with SLE. Lupus nephritis can cause kidney damage or maybe renal failure if left untreated. Early detection and treatment are crucial for preventing long-term damage.

Fever:
Many people with lupus experience unexplained fevers, which are often one among the primary signs that something is wrong. These fevers are usually mild but persistent, and that they could also be a wake-up call of an impending lupus flare.

Hair Loss:
Hair thinning or loss, especially round the temples and along the hairline, is common in lupus. This will be a distressing symptom for patients, as hair loss is usually related to severe disease activity or a flare.

Chest Pain and Shortness of Breath:
Lupus can cause inflammation of the liner round the lungs (pleuritis) or the guts (pericarditis), resulting in pain and difficulty breathing. These symptoms are often alarming, and they require medical attention to rule out other potential causes.

Cognitive Issues:
Some people with lupus experience cognitive dysfunction, often referred to as "lupus fog." This can include problems with memory, concentration, and verbal communication. While not

life-threatening, these cognitive issues are often frustrating and should interfere with daily activities.

Raynaud's Phenomenon:
In lupus patients, Raynaud's phenomenon is common, causing fingers and toes to show white or blue in response to cold or stress. This happens because lupus can affect blood vessels, resulting in reduced blood flow in extremities.

THE CAUSES OF LUPUS

While the precise explanation for lupus remains unclear, researchers believe that a mixture of genetic, environmental, and hormonal factors contributes to its development.

Genetic Factors:
Family history plays a task in lupus, although having a relative with lupus doesn't guarantee that somebody will develop the disease. Studies show that certain genes increase the danger of developing lupus, particularly those involved within the system. However, genetics alone cannot explain why some people develop lupus while others with an equivalent genetic marker don't.

Environmental Triggers:
Environmental factors are thought to trigger lupus in people that are genetically predisposed to the disease. Potential triggers include infections, exposure to ultraviolet (UV) light, and certain medications. While these triggers don't directly cause lupus, they

will activate the system and contribute to disease onset or flare-ups.

Hormonal Influences:

Hormonal factors, particularly estrogen, are believed to play a big role in lupus. This is often one reason why women, especially those of childbearing age, are far more likely to develop lupus than men. Hormonal fluctuations, like people who occur during pregnancy or menopause, also can influence lupus symptoms.

How Lupus Affects the Body

Because lupus may be a systemic disease, it can affect nearly every part of the body. Below are a number of the key organs and systems commonly suffering from lupus.

Skin:

Skin involvement is common in lupus, with rashes, lesions, and sensitivity to sunlight being typical symptoms. These skin issues are often quite cosmetic concerns, as they often signal underlying disease activity.

Joints:

Lupus-related joint pain and swelling are often among the earliest symptoms of the disease. Lupus arthritis is analogous to atrophic arthritis therein it affects multiple joints, but it tends to be less destructive.

Kidneys:

Lupus nephritis may be a serious complication which will cause renal failure if not treated. Early symptoms include swelling within the legs or feet, high vital sign, and changes in urine output or color.

Heart:

Lupus can increase the danger of cardiovascular problems, including heart attacks and strokes. Inflammation of the guts and blood vessels may be a common complication of lupus, and therefore the disease may contribute to the event of atherosclerosis (hardening of the arteries).

Lungs:

Lupus can cause pleurisy (inflammation of the liner round the lungs), which results in pain and difficulty breathing. In rare cases, lupus may cause scarring of the lung tissue

CHAPTER 2

RECOGNIZING THE SYMPTOMS

Lupus presents a singular challenge within the medical world thanks to its wide selection of symptoms, which vary significantly from person to person. The range of symptoms makes it hard for healthcare providers to diagnose and for patients to manage, often leading to delayed diagnosis and treatment. During this chapter, we'll explore the common symptoms of lupus, how they manifest, and why identifying these symptoms early is often so difficult. We'll also check out how these symptoms can overlap with other conditions, adding further complexity to lupus diagnosis and management.

The Nature of Lupus Symptoms

Lupus is often referred to as "the great imitator" because its symptoms mimic those of many other illnesses. Its symptoms can appear gradually or suddenly, and they can range from mild to severe. Some people experience short periods of relatively mild symptoms, while others face long-lasting symptoms which will become life-threatening if not managed properly. One among the foremost distinctive features of lupus is that it can affect multiple organs and systems within the body, including the skin, joints, kidneys, lungs, brain, and heart.

This systemic nature means lupus can present in various ways, often resulting in misdiagnosis or delayed recognition of the disease.

The unpredictable nature of lupus symptoms makes the disease even tougher. Symptoms can come and enter cycles referred to as flares. During a flare, symptoms worsen, often all of sudden, causing sudden physical and emotional distress. After a flare, symptoms may subside for days, weeks, or maybe years, only to reappear unexpectedly. This pattern of remission and relapse can make living with lupus frustrating and exhausting, as patients must constantly adapt to changing conditions.

COMMON SYMPTOMS OF LUPUS

While lupus can affect nearly every part of the body, some symptoms are more common than others. These hallmark symptoms are often the primary sign that something is wrong, though their presence alone might not be enough to point on to lupus. the foremost frequently reported symptoms of lupus include:

Fatigue:
Fatigue is one among the foremost universal symptoms of lupus, affecting an estimated 80-90% of individuals with the disease. Unlike ordinary tiredness, lupus-related fatigue is often overwhelming and protracted, often leaving individuals unable to perform daily activities. It's not uncommon for people with lupus to feel exhausted even after a full night's sleep.

This fatigue can interfere with work, social life, and private relationships, contributing to feelings of frustration and helplessness.

Joint Pain and Stiffness:

Lupus often causes pain, stiffness, and swelling within the joints, particularly within the hands, wrists, and knees. These symptoms resemble those of other sorts of arthritis, like atrophic arthritis, which is why lupus is usually misdiagnosed as arthritis early. Unlike atrophic arthritis, lupus doesn't usually cause long-term joint damage, though the pain is often even debilitating. Joint symptoms tend to be worse within the morning and improve throughout the day, but they will also flare up all of sudden.

Skin Rashes:

One of the most distinctive and recognizable symptoms of lupus is the "butterfly" rash, which appears across the cheeks and nose in about 30% of individuals with the disease. This rash is usually triggered by sun exposure, as many of us with lupus are sensitive to ultraviolet (UV) light. In addition to the butterfly rash, lupus can cause other sorts of skin rashes and lesions, particularly on areas exposed to the sun, like the face, neck, and arms. Discoid lupus, a kind of cutaneous lupus, causes round, raised lesions which will leave scars. These skin issues are often a source of embarrassment and discomfort for several patients, particularly once they occur on visible parts of the body.

Fever:

Many of us with lupus experience unexplained fevers, often between 98.6°F and 100°F. These low-grade fevers are often one among the primary signs of a lupus flare and should occur with or without other symptoms. Because fever may be a symptom of the many common illnesses, it's often overlooked or attributed to infections, which may delay diagnosis.

Hair Loss:

Hair loss or thinning is another common symptom of lupus. The autoimmune response related to lupus can attack the hair follicles, resulting in hair loss on the scalp, eyebrows, and other parts of the body. Hair loss is often temporary, occurring during flares and growing back during remission, or it is often more permanent if scarring occurs on the scalp. These symptoms are often distressing for several patients, because it affects their appearance and self-esteem.

Photosensitivity:

Many of us with lupus are sensitive to sunlight and artificial UV light. Exposure to UV rays can trigger a lupus flare, causing symptoms like skin rashes, joint pain, and fatigue to worsen. Photosensitivity can make it difficult for people with lupus to spend time outdoors or in environments with bright lighting, which may limit their activities and social interactions.

Mouth Sores:

Mouth sores, or ulcers, are a less common but still significant symptom of lupus. These sores can appear on the inside of the mouth, on the lips, or within the nasal passages. they'll be painful or painless, but they're often a symbol of active disease.

Swelling within the Extremities:

Lupus can cause inflammation within the kidneys, resulting in a condition referred to as lupus nephritis. When the kidneys are inflamed, they'll not function properly, leading to the buildup of excess fluid within the body. This will cause swelling within the legs, feet, hands, and round the eyes. Swelling also can occur within the joints, resulting in pain and stiffness.

ORGAN-SPECIFIC SYMPTOMS

One of the defining characteristics of lupus is its ability to affect multiple organs and systems within the body. In addition to the common symptoms described above, lupus can cause more severe and specific symptoms counting on which organs are involved. Below are a number of the foremost critical organ-specific symptoms related to lupus:

Kidney Problems:
Lupus nephritis, or inflammation of the kidneys, is one among the foremost serious complications of lupus. It occurs in about 40-60% of individuals with lupus and may cause permanent kidney damage or maybe renal failure if not treated promptly.

Early symptoms of lupus nephritis include swelling within the legs or feet, high vital sign, and changes in urine output or color (e.g., dark or foamy urine). Because renal disorder often progresses without noticeable symptoms, regular monitoring and blood tests are essential for people with lupus.

Heart and Lung Involvement:
Lupus can affect the circulatory system in several ways, including inflammation of the guts (pericarditis) and lungs (pleuritis). Pericarditis can cause sharp pain, especially when taking deep breaths or lying down. Pleuritis, similarly, causes pain with breathing thanks to inflammation of the liner round the lungs. Lupus also increases the danger of developing blood clots

and atherosclerosis (hardening of the arteries), which may cause heart attacks and strokes. These cardiovascular complications make lupus a big risk factor for heart condition, even in younger individuals.

Brain and systema nervosum Symptoms;
Lupus can affect the brain and central systema nervosum, resulting in a variety of neurological symptoms. Some people with lupus experience headaches, dizziness, memory problems, or difficulty concentrating commonly referred to as "lupus fog." More severe cases of lupus may cause seizures, vision problems, or strokes. In rare instances, lupus can cause psychosis, a mental disturbance during which the individual loses touch with reality. These neurological symptoms are often particularly distressing for patients and their families, as they'll affect cognition, mood, and personality.

Blood and cardiovascular system Issues:
Lupus can affect the blood in several ways, resulting in conditions like anemia, leukopenia (low white blood corpuscle count), and thrombocytopenia (low platelet count). These abnormalities may result in fatigue, increased risk of infection, and straightforward bruising or bleeding. Some people with lupus develop antiphospholipid syndrome (APS), a condition that causes the blood to clot too easily. APS can cause complications like deep vein thrombosis (blood clots within the legs), embolism (blood clots within the lungs), and recurrent miscarriages in pregnant women.

Gastrointestinal Symptoms:

Although less common, lupus can affect the gastrointestinal system, causing symptoms like nausea, vomiting, abdominal pain, and diarrhea. These symptoms could also be associated with inflammation of the alimentary canal or as a side effect of lupus medications.

WHY RECOGNIZING LUPUS SYMPTOMS IS CHALLENGING

One of the foremost challenging aspects of lupus is that its symptoms are often vague, subtle, and simply mistaken for other conditions. Fatigue, joint pain, and rashes are common complaints among people with a good range of illnesses, from the flu to arthritis to skin disorders.

This overlap can make it difficult for both patients and doctors to spot lupus early, resulting in delayed diagnosis and treatment.

Many people with lupus report seeing multiple doctors and receiving various diagnoses before finally being diagnosed with lupus. Because lupus can affect numerous parts of the body, patients often see specialists for specific symptoms, like a dermatologist for rashes, a rheumatologist for joint pain, or a nephrologist for kidney issues. Without a comprehensive view of the patient's health, these specialists might not recognize the underlying explanation for the symptoms.

In some cases, people with lupus may be told that their symptoms are "all in their head" or that they are suffering from stress, anxiety, or depression. The invisible nature of some lupus symptoms, like fatigue or cognitive issues, can make it difficult for patients to elucidate their condition to others, resulting in frustration and feelings of isolation.

The Importance Of Early Diagnosis

Early lupus diagnosis is vital because it allows for timely treatment, which can reduce organ damage and enhance quality of life. Early diagnosis allows doctors to control symptoms before they worsen, lowering the chance of serious complications such as renal or heart problems. With an early diagnosis, patients can begin lifestyle changes and medication sooner, reducing flare-ups and limiting long-term complications. Early intervention also provides patients with skills for understanding and monitoring their illness, which leads to better long-term health outcomes.

CHAPTER 3

THE DIAGNOSIS OF LUPUS

Lupus is one among the foremost difficult diseases to diagnose because its symptoms are both varied and sometimes nonspecific. Early detection is critical to stop irreversible organ damage, yet the method of reaching a diagnosis is typically lengthy and frustrating for patients. This chapter explores the diagnostic journey, including the tools and tests doctors use to verify lupus, the challenges related to differentiating it from other illnesses, and therefore the importance of a correct diagnosis in managing the disease effectively.

THE DIAGNOSTIC JOURNEY

For many people with lupus, the trail to diagnosis is long and crammed with uncertainty. Symptoms like fatigue, joint pain, and skin rashes are common in many other conditions, making it hard to pinpoint lupus because of the cause. Additionally, because lupus symptoms can come and go, some patients may feel relatively well during doctor visits, which may cause misdiagnosis or dismissal of their concerns.

On average, it can take months or maybe years for an individual to be accurately diagnosed with lupus. During this point, patients often see multiple healthcare providers and receive various diagnoses, like fibromyalgia, atrophic arthritis, or chronic fatigue syndrome. Some could also be told that their symptoms are psychological or associated with stress, further delaying appropriate treatment.

Lupus may be a disease that needs a comprehensive view of the patient's health. Since the disease can affect multiple organs and systems, specialists from different fields are often involved within the diagnostic process. A rheumatologist, a doctor who focuses on autoimmune diseases, is usually the key specialist involved in diagnosing and treating lupus. However, dermatologists, nephrologists, neurologists, and cardiologists can also play a task, counting on the patient's symptoms.

SYMPTOMS AS CLUES

Because lupus manifests in many various ways, doctors often believe a mixture of symptoms and tests to form a diagnosis. There's no single test which will definitively diagnose lupus, which makes the method challenging. Instead, doctors use a mixture of clinical criteria and laboratory results to create a case for lupus.

Some of the common symptoms which will lead a doctor to suspect lupus include:

Persistent Fatigue:
 Chronic, unexplained fatigue is one among the hallmark symptoms of lupus. While fatigue is common in many other

conditions, its presence in conjunction with other lupus symptoms can raise suspicion.

Joint Pain and Swelling:
Lupus-related joint pain typically affects multiple joints, particularly within the hands, wrists, and knees. The pain often comes with morning stiffness and should improve throughout the day.

Skin Rashes:
The characteristic butterfly rash across the cheeks and nose may be a classic sign of lupus. Other skin rashes, particularly those triggered by sun exposure, also can point toward lupus.

Fever:
Unexplained fevers, especially when combined with fatigue and joint pain, are often an early wake-up call of lupus.

Hair Loss:
While hair loss is often caused by many factors, patchy hair loss or thinning, particularly round the scalp's perimeter, are often a symbol of lupus.

Kidney Problems:
Symptoms like swelling within the legs, feet, or round the eyes, changes in urine output, or dark, foamy urine may indicate lupus nephritis, a significant complication of lupus.

While these symptoms may suggest lupus, they're not enough to verify the diagnosis on their own. Doctors must believe a mixture of physical examinations, medical records, and laboratory tests to form an accurate diagnosis.

DIAGNOSTIC CRITERIA

The American College of Rheumatology (ACR) and therefore the Systemic Lupus International Collaborating Clinics (SLICC) have established specific criteria to assist doctors diagnose lupus. consistent with these guidelines, an individual must meet a particular number of criteria, either from clinical findings (such as symptoms) or laboratory results, to be diagnosed with lupus. These criteria were developed to standardize the diagnostic process and make sure that doctors consider the wide selection of symptoms and lab abnormalities related to lupus.

The ACR and SLICC criteria include:

1. Skin and Mucous Membranes:
This includes the butterfly rash, discoid rash (round, raised patches of skin), and photosensitivity (rashes triggered by sun exposure).

2. Joint Involvement:
Pain, stiffness, and swelling in two or more joints, particularly without significant joint damage.

3. Kidney Involvement:
Protein within the urine (proteinuria) or abnormal kidney function tests, which can indicate lupus nephritis.

4. Serositis:

Inflammation of the liner round the heart (pericarditis) or lungs (pleuritis), which causes pain, particularly with deep breathing.

5. Neurological Symptoms:

Seizures, psychosis, or cognitive dysfunction can point to central systema nervosum involvement in lupus.

6. Blood Abnormalities:

Low red blood corpuscle count (anemia), low white blood corpuscle count (leukopenia), or low platelet count (thrombocytopenia) are common in lupus.

7. Immunological Markers:

The presence of specific autoantibodies, like anti-dsDNA, anti-Sm, and antiphospholipid antibodies, can help confirm lupus.

8. Antinuclear Antibodies (ANA):

A positive ANA test is present in nearly all people with lupus, though a positive result alone doesn't confirm the diagnosis, as ANA are often positive in other autoimmune diseases and even in healthy individuals.

According to the standards, an individual is often diagnosed with lupus if they meet a minimum of four of the clinical and immunological criteria, with a minimum of one clinical and one immunological criterion. This approach helps doctors identify lupus even when its symptoms are subtle or overlap with other conditions.

LABORATORY TESTS UTILIZED IN DIAGNOSIS

In addition to clinical criteria, doctors use a spread of laboratory tests to assist diagnose lupus. These tests can provide important information about how the disease affects the body and help rule out other conditions with similar symptoms. a number of the foremost commonly used tests within the diagnosis of lupus include:

Antinuclear Antibody (ANA) Test:

The ANA test is one among the foremost important tests utilized in diagnosing lupus. ANA are antibodies that focus on the nuclei of the body's cells. A positive ANA test indicates that the system is producing autoantibodies, which is common in lupus and other autoimmune diseases. However, a positive ANA test alone doesn't confirm lupus, because it is often positive in other conditions or maybe in healthy individuals. If the ANA test is positive, additional tests could also be conducted to see for specific autoantibodies related to lupus.

Anti-dsDNA Test:

This test detects antibodies to double-stranded DNA, which are highly specific to lupus. A positive anti-dsDNA test strongly suggests lupus, particularly if the person has other symptoms of the disease. High levels of anti-dsDNA antibodies are often related to lupus nephritis and more severe disease.

Anti-Smith (Anti-Sm) Test:

Anti-Sm antibodies are another sort of autoantibody that's specific to lupus. While only about 20-30% of individuals with lupus have these antibodies, their presence may be a strong indicator of the disease.

Antiphospholipid Antibody Test:
Antiphospholipid antibodies are related to an increased risk of blood clots and recurrent miscarriages in people with lupus. Testing for these antibodies is vital for identifying potential complications and guiding treatment decisions.

Complement Levels:
Complement proteins are a part of the system that helps fight infections. In people with lupus, complement levels (particularly C3 and C4) could also be low, indicating that the system is overly active and consumes these proteins.

Complete Blood Count (CBC):
A CBC measures the amount of red blood cells, white blood cells, and platelets. Abnormalities in these levels can suggest lupus, particularly if the person has anemia, leukopenia, or thrombocytopenia.

Urinalysis:
A urinalysis checks for the presence of protein or blood within the urine, which may indicate kidney damage or lupus nephritis.

Erythrocyte erythrocyte sedimentation rate (ESR) and C-reactive protein (CRP):
Both ESR and CRP are markers of inflammation within the body. While these tests aren't specific to lupus, elevated levels may indicate active inflammation and help doctors monitor disease activity.

IMAGING AND BIOPSY

In some cases, doctors may use imaging studies or biopsies to assist diagnose lupus, particularly if the disease affects specific organs.

Kidney Biopsy:
A kidney biopsy involves removing a little sample of kidney tissue for examination under a microscope. This test is usually wont to diagnose lupus nephritis and determine the severity of kidney damage.

Chest X-ray or CT Scan:
If lupus is suspected to be affecting the lungs or heart, a chest X-ray or CT scan can help detect inflammation or fluid buildup within the lungs (pleuritis) or round the heart (pericarditis).

Echocardiogram:
An echocardiogram is an ultrasound of the guts which will detect inflammation, fluid buildup, or other abnormalities within the heart caused by lupus.

DIFFERENTIATING LUPUS FROM OTHER CONDITIONS

One of the foremost significant challenges in diagnosing lupus is differentiating it from other conditions with similar symptoms. Because lupus affects multiple systems within the body, its symptoms often overlap with those of other autoimmune diseases, like atrophic arthritis, scleroderma, or Sjogren's syndrome. Additionally, conditions like fibromyalgia, chronic fatigue syndrome, and even certain infections can mimic lupus symptoms, making it difficult to pinpoint the correct diagnosis.

Doctors must carefully consider the patient's medical record, symptoms, and test results to rule out other conditions and ensure lupus. This process often takes time and should involve seeing multiple specialists before a diagnosis is reached.

THE ROLE OF THE PATIENT IN DIAGNOSIS

Patients play an important role within the diagnostic process. Because lupus symptoms can vary widely from person to person, it's important for patients to stay track of their symptoms and share this information with their doctor. Keeping a symbol diary is often helpful in identifying patterns, like when symptoms worsen or improve, what triggers flares, and the way symptoms affect lifestyle.

Patients should also advocate for themselves during the diagnostic process. If a doctor dismisses symptoms or provides a diagnosis that doesn't seem to suit, it's important to hunt a second opinion or invite further testing. Early diagnosis is critical in lupus, because it allows for prompt treatment which will prevent organ damage and improve quality of life.

The Importance of an Accurate Diagnosis

An accurate diagnosis of lupus is important for effective treatment and management of the disease. Without a correct diagnosis, patients might not receive the treatment they have to regulate their symptoms and stop complications. In some cases, misdiagnosis can cause inappropriate treatments which will worsen the condition or cause unnecessary side effects.

Once a diagnosis of lupus is confirmed, patients can begin working with their healthcare team to develop a customized treatment plan. This plan may include medications to regulate inflammation and stop organ damage, lifestyle changes to scale back symptoms and improve overall health, and regular monitoring to detect and treat complications early.

An accurate diagnosis also provides patients with validation and understanding. Many of us with lupus experience years of uncertainty and frustration as they look for answers to their symptoms.

A confirmed diagnosis can provide relief, because it gives patients a reputation for his or her condition and allows them to attach with resources, support groups, et al. living with lupus.

In the next chapter, we'll delve into the varied treatment options available for managing lupus, including medications, lifestyle changes, and alternative therapies.

CHAPTER 4

TREATMENT AND MANAGEMENT OF LUPUS

The management of lupus requires a multifaceted approach thanks to the complexity and variability of the disease. Effective treatment aims to regulate symptoms, prevent flares, and reduce the danger of complications. This chapter will explore the varied treatment options available for lupus, including medications, lifestyle modifications, and complementary therapies. Understanding these options can help patients work with their healthcare team to develop a customized plan that most accurately fits their needs.

PHARMACOLOGICAL TREATMENTS

Medications play a central role in managing lupus. The selection of medication depends on the severity of the disease, the organs affected, and therefore the patient's overall health. The most categories of medicines wont to treat lupus include nonsteroidal anti-inflammatory drug drugs (NSAIDs), antimalarials, corticosteroids, immunosuppressives, and biologics.

Nonsteroidal Anti-Inflammatory Drugs (NSAIDs):
 NSAIDs are often wont to manage mild to moderate symptoms of lupus, like joint pain, muscle aches, and fevers. These drugs

work by reducing inflammation and pain. Common NSAIDs include ibuprofen, naproxen, and aspirin. While effective for symptom relief, long-term use of NSAIDs can cause gastrointestinal issues, kidney problems, and cardiovascular risks, in order that they should be used with caution and under medical supervision.

Antimalarials:

Hydroxychloroquine (Plaquenil) is an antimalarial that has become a cornerstone of lupus treatment. It helps control skin rashes, joint pain, and fatigue, and should reduce the frequency of disease flares. Antimalarials are generally well-tolerated but can cause side effects like nausea, diarrhea, and visual disturbances in some patients. Regular eye exams are recommended to watch for potential retinal damage.

Corticosteroids:

Corticosteroids, like prednisone, are powerful anti-inflammatory drugs wont to manage acute flares of lupus and severe symptoms. They work by suppressing the immune system's activity, reducing inflammation and swelling. While effective, long-term use of corticosteroids can cause significant side effects, including weight gain, osteoporosis, diabetes, and hypertension. Doctors aim to use rock bottom effective doses for the shortest period necessary to attenuate these risks.

Immunosuppressives:

Immunosuppressive drugs, like azathioprine (Imuran), methotrexate, and mycophenolate mofetil (CellCept), are wont to suppress the overactive immune reaction in lupus. These medications are often prescribed when corticosteroids alone are insufficient or when there's significant organ involvement, like lupus nephritis. Immunosuppressives can help control disease activity and stop damage to organs but may increase the danger of infections and certain cancers. Regular blood tests are required to watch for potential side effects.

Biologics:

Biologic drugs, like belimumab (Benlysta) and rituximab (Rituxan), target specific components of the system involved in lupus. Belimumab inhibits a protein called B-lymphocyte stimulator (BLyS) that helps B cells produce autoantibodies. Rituximab targets and depletes B cells that produce these autoantibodies. Biologics are typically used for patients with moderate to severe lupus who don't answer conventional treatments. they will be effective in reducing disease activity and improving quality of life but may have risks like infusion reactions and infections.

LIFESTYLE MODIFICATIONS

In addition to medications, lifestyle modifications are crucial in managing lupus. These changes can help reduce symptoms, improve overall health, and enhance the standard of life. Key lifestyle modifications include:

Sun Protection:

Many of us with lupus are sensitive to sunlight, which may trigger skin rashes and flares. To guard ourselves, individuals should use sunscreen with a high SPF, wear protective clothing, and avoid direct sun exposure, especially during peak hours. Sun protection can help manage skin symptoms and reduce the danger of flare-ups.

Healthy Diet:

A diet is vital for managing lupus and maintaining overall health. A diet rich in fruits, vegetables, whole grains, lean proteins, and healthy fats can help support the system and reduce inflammation. Some people with lupus may have to avoid certain foods or follow specific dietary guidelines supporting their symptoms or related health issues, like high vital signs or kidney problems.

Regular Exercise:

Regular physical activity can help manage lupus symptoms by improving mood, reducing fatigue, and maintaining joint flexibility. Low-impact exercises, like swimming, walking, and yoga, are generally recommended to avoid putting an excessive amount of strain on the joints. It's important for people with lupus to figure with their healthcare provider to develop an exercise plan that suits their condition and fitness level.

Stress Management:

Stress can exacerbate lupus symptoms and trigger flares. Techniques for managing stress include relaxation exercises, mindfulness, meditation, and therapy. Stress management can help improve emotional well-being and overall health.

Adequate Rest:

Rest is important for managing fatigue and allowing the body to get over the consequences of lupus. Patients should aim for normal, restorative sleep and hear their bodies once they get to rest. Establishing a uniform sleep routine and creating a soothing bedtime environment also can help improve sleep quality.

MONITORING AND FOLLOW-UP CARE

Ongoing monitoring and follow-up care are critical components of lupus management. Regular check-ups with a healthcare provider help track disease activity, monitor for complications, and adjust treatment as required. Key aspects of monitoring include:

Regular Lab Tests:
Routine laboratory tests are wont to monitor disease activity and therefore the effects of medicines. Common tests include blood tests to see for anemia, kidney function, and levels of autoantibodies, also as urinalysis to detect changes in kidney function.

Imaging Studies:
Periodic imaging studies, like chest X-rays or ultrasounds, could also be used to monitor the condition of specific organs suffering from lupus, like the guts or kidneys.

Specialist Visits:
counting on the organs suffering from lupus, patients may have to ascertain specialists, like nephrologists for kidney involvement, dermatologists for skin issues, or cardiologists for heart problems. Coordinating care among specialists ensures a comprehensive approach to managing lupus.

Adjusting Treatment:

Treatment plans may have to be adjusted to support changes in disease activity, side effects of medicines, or the event of latest symptoms. Regular follow-up visits provide a chance to assess the effectiveness of the treatment plan and make necessary changes.

COMPLEMENTARY THERAPIES

Some people with lupus explore complementary therapies to assist manage their symptoms and improve their overall well-being. These therapies are used alongside conventional medical treatments and will be discussed with a healthcare provider to make sure they're safe and effective. Common complementary therapies include:

Acupuncture:

Acupuncture involves inserting thin needles into specific points on the body to assist relieve pain and improve overall health. Some people with lupus find that acupuncture helps reduce joint pain and improve energy levels.

Massage Therapy:

Massage therapy can help alleviate muscle tension, improve circulation, and reduce stress. It's going to be beneficial for managing pain and stiffness in individuals with lupus, though it's important to settle on a professional therapist who understands the requirements of individuals with chronic conditions.

Herbal Supplements:

Certain herbal supplements, like turmeric or ginger, are thought to possess anti-inflammatory properties which will benefit people with lupus. However, it's essential to consult a healthcare provider before starting any new supplements, as they'll interact with medications or have potential side effects.

Mind-Body Practices:
Techniques like yoga, tai chi, and mindfulness meditation can help manage stress, improve flexibility, and enhance overall well-being. These practices are often tailored to accommodate physical limitations and individual preferences.

PATIENT EDUCATION AND SUPPORT

Education and support are vital components of lupus management. Understanding the disease, its treatment options, and the way to manage symptoms empowers patients to require a lively role in their care. Support groups and academic resources can provide valuable information, encouragement, and a way of community.

Patient Education:
Learning about lupus, its symptoms, and treatment options helps patients make informed decisions about their care. Educational materials, workshops, and counseling can provide valuable information and support.

Support Groups:

Support groups offer a secure space for people with lupus to share their experiences, gain emotional support, and learn from others who understand the challenges of living with the disease. Connecting with others who have similar experiences can provide practical advice, encouragement, and a way of camaraderie.

Mental Health Support:
Dealing with a chronic illness like lupus are often emotionally challenging. Psychological state support, including counseling or therapy, can help patients manage the psychological impact of the disease and improve their overall well-being.

LIVING WITH LUPUS

Living with lupus requires ongoing management and adaptation. The disease is often unpredictable, and patients must navigate its challenges while maintaining their overall health and quality of life. With a comprehensive treatment plan, lifestyle modifications, and a robust support network, individuals with lupus can lead fulfilling and active lives.

In the next chapter, we'll explore the impact of lupus on lifestyle, including its effects on work, relationships, and psychological state. Understanding these aspects can provide valuable insights into how lupus affects individuals and their families, and offer strategies for dealing with its challenges.

CHAPTER 5

LIVING WITH LUPUS

Lupus isn't just a medical condition; it profoundly affects many aspects of lifestyle. The unpredictability of the disease, combined with its wide-ranging symptoms, can impact work, relationships, psychological state, and overall quality of life. This chapter will explore how lupus influences these areas and offer practical strategies for managing its effects.

IMPACT ON WORK

For many individuals with lupus, maintaining employment is often challenging. The disease's symptoms, like fatigue, joint pain, and cognitive difficulties, can interfere with work performance and attendance. Additionally, frequent medical appointments and therefore the need for infrequent leave can disrupt a person's career.

Managing Symptoms at Work:
 Finding ways to manage symptoms while working is crucial. Strategies include:

Flexible Work Arrangements:
 If possible, discuss flexible work arrangements together with your employer, like telecommuting or adjusted work hours. This

flexibility can help accommodate fluctuating symptoms and reduce stress.

Ergonomic Adjustments:

Adjusting your workspace to enhance ergonomics can help manage joint pain and fatigue. Use supportive chairs, adjustable desks, and ergonomic tools to scale back physical strain.

Breaks and Rest:

Regular breaks can help manage fatigue and stop burnout. Short breaks throughout the day, alongside periodic rest, can help maintain productivity and luxury.

Job Accommodations:

In some cases, it's going to be necessary to request job accommodations under the Americans with Disabilities Act (ADA). This might include adjustments to job responsibilities, work environment, or scheduling to assist manage symptoms.

Communicating with Employers:

Open communication together with your employer is vital to managing lupus within the workplace. Discuss your needs and limitations candidly, and explore possible accommodations or adjustments that would assist you perform your job effectively.

Career Planning:

Consider career planning and development in light of your health. you'll have to explore different career paths or job roles that better align together with your energy levels and physical capabilities.

IMPACT ON RELATIONSHIPS

Lupus can affect relationships with family, friends, and partners thanks to its physical and emotional impact. Understanding and managing these effects can help maintain healthy and supportive relationships.

Family Dynamics:

relations may have to regulate the stress of living with lupus. Open communication about your needs, limitations, and the way the disease affects you'll help relations understand and supply support. It's also important to debate ways to share responsibilities and find balance within the family dynamic.

Friendships:

Friends might not always understand the challenges of living with lupus, especially if symptoms aren't visible. Educating friends about the disease and the way it affects you'll help foster empathy and support. It's also important to take care of connections and have interaction in social activities that you simply enjoy and may manage.

Romantic Relationships:

Lupus can affect romantic relationships in various ways, including physical intimacy and emotional connection. Open and honest communication together with your partner about your condition, treatment, and the way it impacts your relationship is important. Seeking couples counseling or support also can help address any challenges that arise.

Support Networks:

Building a support network of people who understand your experience with lupus can provide emotional support and practical advice. Support groups, both in-person and online, offer a way of community and shared experience.

IMPACT ON MENTAL HEALTH

Living with a chronic illness like lupus can take a toll on psychological state. The strain of managing symptoms, handling uncertainty, and dealing with the impact on lifestyle can cause feelings of depression, anxiety, and frustration.

Recognizing psychological state Challenges:
It's important to acknowledge the signs of psychological state challenges, like persistent sadness, anxiety, difficulty concentrating, or loss of interest in activities. Addressing these symptoms early can help prevent them from becoming more severe.

Seeking Professional Help:
psychological state professionals, like therapists or counselors, can provide valuable support in managing the emotional impact of lupus. Cognitive-behavioral therapy (CBT) and other therapeutic approaches can help individuals develop coping strategies and address negative thought patterns.

Stress Management:
Managing stress is crucial for mental well-being. Techniques like mindfulness, relaxation exercises, and stress management strategies can help reduce the emotional burden of living with

lupus. Incorporating activities that bring joy and relaxation into your routine also can be beneficial.

Support Groups:

Participating in support groups for people with lupus can provide a way of belonging and reduce feelings of isolation. Sharing experiences with others who understand the challenges of living with lupus offers comfort and practical advice.

MANAGING DAILY LIFE

Managing lifestyle with lupus involves adapting to the disease's impact and finding strategies to take care of an honest quality of life. This includes managing symptoms, balancing responsibilities, and maintaining a positive outlook.

Daily Routine Adjustments:

Adjusting your daily routine to accommodate symptoms can help manage fatigue and improve overall well-being. Prioritize tasks, break them into smaller steps, and incorporate rest periods throughout the day.

Self-Care Practices:

Engaging in self-care practices is important for managing lupus and maintaining overall health. This includes following a healthy diet, getting regular exercise, practicing stress management techniques, and ensuring adequate rest.

Setting Realistic Goals:

Set realistic goals for yourself that support your energy levels and capabilities. Break larger goals into smaller, manageable steps and celebrate achievements along the way.

Seeking Assistance:
Don't hesitate to hunt for assistance when needed. Whether it's help with household chores, transportation to medical appointments, or emotional support, reaching out for help can ease the burden and improve your quality of life.

Staying Informed:
Stay informed about lupus and its management. Knowledge about the disease, treatment options, and new research can empower you to form informed decisions and advocate for your health.

LIVING WITH HOPE

While lupus presents significant challenges, many individuals with the disease lead fulfilling and active lives. Advances in research, treatment options, and supportive care still improve outcomes and quality of life for people with lupus.

Embracing a Positive Outlook:
Maintaining a positive outlook and specializing in what you'll control can help improve your overall well-being. Celebrate successes, practice gratitude, and find joy in lifestyle.

Connecting with Others:
Building connections with others who have lupus and participating in support networks can provide encouragement and shared experiences. These connections offer valuable insights and support.

Advocacy and Awareness:

Advocating for lupus awareness and supporting research can contribute to progress within the field and improve the lives of these suffering from the disease. Engaging in advocacy efforts can provide a way of purpose and contribute to positive change.

In the next chapter, we'll delve into the long-term outlook for people with lupus, including considerations for disease progression, management of complications, and methods for maintaining health and well-being over the years. Understanding the long-term aspects of lupus can help patients plan for the longer term and navigate the continued challenges of living with the disease.

CHAPTER 6

THE LONG-TERM OUTLOOK FOR LUPUS

Lupus may be a chronic condition that needs ongoing management and monitoring. Understanding the long-term outlook for lupus involves considering how the disease progresses, managing potential complications, and maintaining overall health and well-being. This chapter will explore these aspects and offer strategies for navigating the long-term journey with lupus.

DISEASE PROGRESSION

Lupus is characterized by periods of flares and remission, and its progression can vary significantly from person to person. Some individuals experience mild symptoms with few complications, while others may face more severe manifestations affecting multiple organs.

Patterns of Disease Activity:
Lupus can present with fluctuating disease activity. Some individuals may have well-controlled symptoms with long periods of remission, while others experience frequent flares.

Regular monitoring and adjustment of treatment are crucial for managing disease activity and preventing complications.

Organ Involvement:
Lupus can affect various organs, including the skin, joints, kidneys, heart, and lungs. The extent of organ involvement can influence the long-term outlook. for instance, lupus nephritis (kidney involvement) requires careful management to stop kidney damage, while cardiac involvement may necessitate ongoing cardiovascular care.

Predicting Disease Course:
Predicting the course of lupus is often challenging thanks to its variability. Some factors, like early diagnosis, prompt treatment, and adherence to management strategies, can positively impact the long-term outlook. Regular follow-ups and monitoring are essential to adapt treatment plans to support disease progression.

MANAGING COMPLICATIONS

Long-term management of lupus involves addressing and preventing complications which will arise thanks to the disease or its treatments.

Kidney Complications:
Lupus nephritis can cause chronic renal disorder or renal failure if not managed effectively. Regular monitoring of kidney function through blood tests and urinalysis is vital. Treatment may include medications to regulate inflammation and reduce

proteinuria (excess protein within the urine). In severe cases, dialysis or kidney transplantation could also be necessary.

Cardiovascular Health:
People with lupus are at increased risk of cardiovascular issues, including heart condition and stroke. Managing risk factors like high vital signs, high cholesterol, and diabetes is crucial. A heart-healthy lifestyle, including regular exercise and a diet, can help reduce cardiovascular risk.

Bone Health:
Long-term use of corticosteroids can cause osteoporosis and increased risk of fractures. Patients should discuss bone health with their healthcare provider and should take medications or supplements to strengthen bones. Weight-bearing exercises and a diet rich in calcium and vitamin D also can support bone health.

Infections:
Immunosuppressive medications can increase susceptibility to infections. It's important to require preventive measures, like vaccinations and practicing good hygiene. Prompt treatment of infections and regular monitoring for signs of illness are essential for managing infection risk.

Mental Health:
Chronic illness can impact psychological state, resulting in stress, anxiety, or depression. Addressing psychological state needs through counseling, support groups, and stress management techniques can improve overall well-being and quality of life.

MAINTAINING HEALTH AND WELL-BEING

Maintaining health and well-being over the future involves a proactive approach to self-care and disease management.

Regular Medical Check-ups:

Routine medical check-ups are essential for monitoring disease activity, assessing treatment effectiveness, and detecting potential complications early. Regular visits with a rheumatologist and other specialists as required help ensure comprehensive care.

Adherence to Treatment:

Adhering to prescribed treatments and medications is crucial for managing lupus and preventing complications. Communicate together with your healthcare team about any side effects or concerns with medications, and work together to seek out effective solutions.

Healthy Lifestyle Choices:

Adopting a healthy lifestyle supports overall well-being and helps manage lupus. Key components include:

Balanced Diet:

A nutritious diet supports immune function, reduces inflammation, and maintains overall health. specialize in whole foods, including fruits, vegetables, lean proteins, and whole grains.

Regular Exercise:

Engaging in regular physical activity can improve cardiovascular health, manage weight, and reduce stress. Choose low-impact exercises that are gentle on the joints, like walking, swimming, or yoga.

Adequate Sleep:

Quality sleep is important for managing fatigue and supporting overall health. Establish a uniform sleep routine and make a restful sleep environment.

Stress Management:

Managing stress through relaxation techniques, mindfulness, and hobbies can improve psychological state and reduce the impact of lupus symptoms. Incorporate stress-reducing activities into your daily routine.

Support Systems:

Building and maintaining a robust network is vital for emotional well-being. Connect with family, friends, and support groups to share experiences, seek advice, and receive encouragement.

ADVANCEMENTS IN RESEARCH AND TREATMENT

Ongoing research continues to advance the understanding of lupus and improve treatment options. Staying informed about new developments offers hope and potential benefits for managing the disease.

Emerging Therapies:

Advances in research may cause new therapies and treatment options for lupus. Stay informed about clinical trials, new medications, and innovative approaches to disease management.

Personalized Medicine:

Personalized medicine aims to tailor treatments supporting individual patient characteristics, including genetic and environmental factors. This approach has the potential to enhance treatment outcomes and minimize side effects.

Patient Advocacy:

Engaging in patient advocacy and supporting lupus research can contribute to progress within the field. Participating in advocacy efforts, fundraising, and raising awareness can help drive positive change and improve outcomes for people with lupus.

Planning for the Future

Planning for the longer term involves considering both the challenges and opportunities which will arise with lupus. This includes:

Long-Term Goals:

Set realistic long-term goals for private and professional aspirations. Work together with your healthcare team to develop strategies for managing lupus while pursuing these goals.

Future Health Considerations:
Anticipate potential health needs and plan accordingly. This might include discussing long-term care options, financial planning, and advance directives together with your healthcare provider and loved ones.

Staying Positive:
Maintaining a positive outlook and that specialize in what you'll control can assist you navigate the long-term journey with lupus. Embrace a proactive approach to self-care and disease management, and seek support when needed.

In the next chapter, we'll explore the role of support systems and resources in managing lupus. Understanding the available support and resources can provide valuable tools and assistance for navigating the challenges of living with lupus and enhancing overall quality of life.

CHAPTER 7

SUPPORT SYSTEMS AND RESOURCES FOR LUPUS

Living with lupus requires quite just medical management; it also involves leveraging support systems and resources to navigate the challenges of the disease. Support systems can provide emotional, practical, and informational assistance, while resources offer tools and guidance for managing lupus effectively. This chapter will explore various support systems and resources available to individuals with lupus and their families.

SUPPORT SYSTEMS

Support systems play an important role in helping individuals with lupus deal with the emotional and practical aspects of the disease. Building a robust support network can provide comfort, encouragement, and practical help.

Family and Friends:
Family and friends are often the first sources of support for people with lupus. Open communication about the disease, its impact, and your needs can help family and friends provide appropriate support. Educating loved ones about lupus can foster

empathy and understanding, enabling them to supply simpler assistance.

Educational Resources:

Providing educational materials or directing loved ones to reputable resources can help them understand lupus better. This will include information on managing symptoms, the impact of the disease, and ways to supply support.

Involvement in Care:

 relations and friends can assist with daily tasks, medical appointments, and emotional support. Involving them in your care plan can help make sure that you've got the support you would like to manage your condition effectively.

Support Groups:

Support groups offer a community of people who understand the unique challenges of living with lupus. These groups can provide a way of belonging, practical advice, and emotional support.

In-Person Support Groups:

Many communities have local lupus support groups that meet regularly. These groups often offer opportunities for people to share experiences, discuss coping strategies, and receive support from others with similar experiences.

Online Support Groups:

Online support groups and forums provide access to a wider network of people with lupus. They provide the ability to attach from home and participate in discussions at any time. Online groups also can be a valuable resource for locating information and sharing experiences with a broader audience.

Counseling and Therapy:
Professional counseling and therapy can provide additional support for managing the emotional impact of lupus. Therapists and counselors can help individuals deal with stress, anxiety, and depression related to chronic illness.

Cognitive-Behavioral Therapy (CBT):
CBT may be a common therapeutic approach which will help individuals address negative thought patterns and develop coping strategies. It is often particularly useful for managing the psychological impact of living with lupus.

Family Therapy:
Group therapy can help address relationship dynamics suffering from lupus and improve communication and support within the family. It is often beneficial for navigating the challenges that the disease brings to family life.

MEDICAL AND HEALTH RESOURCES

Medical and health resources provide essential information and tools for managing lupus. These resources can help individuals stay informed about their condition, access treatment, and make informed decisions about their care.

Healthcare Providers:

Building a robust relationship with a healthcare provider is prime to effective lupus management. Rheumatologists, medical care doctors, and specialists play key roles in diagnosing and treating lupus, monitoring disease activity, and adjusting treatment plans.

Specialist Care:
counting on the extent of organ involvement, individuals with lupus may have to ascertain specialists like nephrologists, dermatologists, cardiologists, or pulmonologists. Coordinating care among specialists ensures comprehensive management of the disease.

Patient Portals:
Many healthcare systems offer patient portals that provide access to medical records, test results, and communication with healthcare providers. Utilizing these portals can help individuals stay informed about their health and manage their care effectively.

Educational Websites and Resources:
Reliable educational websites offer information on lupus, its management, and research advancements. These resources can help individuals understand their condition and make informed decisions about their care.

Lupus Organizations:
National and native lupus organizations, like the Lupus Foundation of America and therefore the Lupus Research Alliance, provide educational materials, support services, and advocacy efforts. These organizations often offer resources like brochures, webinars, and informational articles.

Medical Journals and Research:

Accessing medical journals and research articles can provide insights into the newest developments in lupus treatment and management. Consulting with healthcare providers about relevant research can help individuals stay up-to-date with advancements within the field.

FINANCIAL AND PRACTICAL ASSISTANCE

Managing lupus can involve significant financial and practical challenges. Accessing financial assistance and practical support can help alleviate a number of these burdens.

Insurance and Financial Assistance:

Navigating coverage and financial assistance options is crucial for managing the prices related to lupus treatment. Understanding insurance benefits, copayments, and out-of-pocket expenses can help individuals plan and allow their care.

Patient Assistance Programs:

Many pharmaceutical companies offer patient assistance programs that provide support or discounted medications for eligible individuals. Contacting drug manufacturers or patient advocacy organizations can help identify available programs.

Government Programs:

Government programs like Social Security social insurance (SSDI) and Supplemental Security Income (SSI) may provide support for people who are unable to figure thanks to their condition. Researching eligibility and application processes can help access these resources.

Practical Support Services:
Practical support services can assist with daily tasks and responsibilities. These services may include:

Home Care Services:
Home care services can provide assistance with activities of daily living, like care, housekeeping, and meal preparation. These services are often particularly helpful for people with severe symptoms or mobility issues.

Transportation Services:
Transportation services can assist with going to medical appointments, grocery shopping, and other errands. Many communities offer transportation programs for people with disabilities or chronic illnesses.

Legal and Advocacy Services:
Legal and advocacy services can provide support with issues like employment discrimination, disability rights, and access to healthcare. Organizations specializing in disability law offer guidance and assistance.

EDUCATION AND ADVOCACY

Education and advocacy play vital roles in improving the lives of people with lupus. Engaging in advocacy efforts and educating others about the disease can help drive progress and increase awareness.

Advocacy Efforts:
Participating in advocacy efforts can contribute to positive change in lupus research, treatment, and policy. Advocacy organizations and campaigns work to boost awareness, support research funding, and promote policy changes that benefit individuals with lupus.

Volunteering and Fundraising:
Volunteering with lupus organizations and participating in fundraising events can support research and lift awareness about the disease. These efforts help drive progress and supply valuable resources for people with lupus.

Policy Engagement:
Engaging with policymakers and advocating for healthcare policies that benefit individuals with lupus can cause improvements in access to worry and support services. Staying informed about policy issues and participating in advocacy campaigns can make a difference.

Educational Outreach:
Educating the general public and healthcare professionals about lupus can improve understanding and reduce stigma. Sharing personal experiences, participating in educational events, and providing information about the disease can help increase awareness and support.

BUILDING A SUPPORTIVE COMMUNITY

Creating a supportive community involves connecting with others who share similar experiences and fostering a network of support. Building and participating during a community can enhance overall well-being and supply valuable resources.

Online Communities:

Online communities and forums offer a platform for connecting with others living with lupus. These communities provide opportunities for sharing experiences, seeking advice, and offering support.

Local and National Events:

Attending local and national lupus events, like conferences, workshops, and support group meetings, can provide opportunities for learning, networking, and connecting with others.

Peer Support:

Peer support, including mentorship and buddy systems, offers personalized guidance and encouragement. Connecting with others who have similar experiences can provide valuable insights and emotional support.

In the next chapter, we'll explore the longer term of lupus research and advancements in treatment. Understanding the newest developments and potential breakthroughs offers hope and informs strategies for managing lupus and improving quality of life.

CHAPTER 8

WAY FORWARD FOR LUPUS RESEARCH AND ADVANCEMENTS IN TREATMENT

The field of lupus research is dynamic, with ongoing advancements that promise to rework the way we understand and treat this complex disease. This chapter explores the present state of lupus research, emerging treatments, and future directions which will enhance disease management and improve patient outcomes.

CURRENT RESEARCH LANDSCAPE

Lupus research encompasses a good range of studies aimed toward understanding the disease, identifying biomarkers, and developing new treatments. Research efforts specialize in various aspects of lupus, including its causes, mechanisms, and potential therapeutic targets.

Understanding Disease Mechanisms:
 Researchers are investigating the underlying mechanisms that drive lupus. Studies specialize in the immune system's role within the disease, including how it mistakenly attacks healthy

tissues. Advances in genetics, genomics, and proteomics are providing insights into the molecular pathways involved in lupus.

Genetic Research:

Genetic studies aim to spot specific genes related to lupus and understand their role in disease development. Identifying genetic risk factors can help in predicting disease susceptibility and tailoring personalized treatment approaches.

Immunological Studies:

Immunological research explores the immune system's abnormalities in lupus, like the role of autoantibodies and immune cell dysfunction. Understanding these mechanisms can cause targeted therapies that address the basic causes of disease activity.

Biomarker Discovery:

Biomarkers are indicators which will help diagnose lupus, predict disease activity, and monitor treatment response. Researchers are developing and validating biomarkers that would cause earlier diagnosis and more personalized treatment strategies.

Diagnostic Biomarkers:

Identifying biomarkers which will differentiate lupus from other autoimmune diseases is crucial for accurate diagnosis. Research is concentrated on finding reliable biomarkers that reflect disease activity and progression.

Predictive Biomarkers:

Predictive biomarkers aim to spot individuals in danger of severe disease or complications. These biomarkers could guide early interventions and preventive measures to enhance long-term outcomes.

EMERGING TREATMENTS

Recent advances in treatment research have led to the development of the latest therapies that provide hope for better disease management and improved quality of life. These treatments target specific aspects of lupus and aim to scale back disease activity and stop complications.

Biologic Therapies:

Biologics are a category of medicine that focus on specific molecules or cells involved within the disease process. Several biologics are approved or are in development for lupus.

B-Cell Targeted Therapies:

B-cell targeted therapies, like belimumab (Benlysta), specialize in inhibiting B-cells, which play a central role in lupus. These therapies have shown promise in reducing disease activity and improving patient outcomes.

T-Cell Targeted Therapies:

T-cell targeted therapies aim to modulate the activity of T-cells, which are involved in autoimmune responses. Research is exploring drugs that specifically target T-cell activation or function to scale back inflammation and tissue damage.

Interleukin Inhibitors:

Interleukins are cytokines involved within the immune reaction. Inhibitors of specific interleukins, like interleukin-6 (IL-6) and interleukin-1 (IL-1), are being studied for his or her potential to scale back inflammation and disease activity in lupus.

Targeted Small Molecule Drugs:

Targeted small molecules are designed to interfere with specific pathways involved in lupus. These drugs may offer oral administration options and supply new treatment avenues.

Janus Kinase (JAK) Inhibitors:

JAK inhibitors, like tofacitinib, target enzymes involved in inflammatory signaling pathways. These drugs have shown efficacy in treating other autoimmune diseases and are being investigated for his or her potential benefits in lupus.

Sphingosine-1-Phosphate (S1P) Receptor Modulators:

S1P receptor modulators are being explored for his or her ability to modulate immune cell migration and reduce inflammation. These drugs have the potential to supply new treatment options for lupus patients.

Combination Therapies:

Combining different treatments may enhance efficacy and reduce side effects. Research is exploring combination therapies that integrate biologics, targeted small molecules, and traditional drugs to supply simpler and personalized treatment strategies.

PERSONALIZED MEDICINE

Personalized medicine aims to tailor treatments supporting individual patient characteristics, including genetic, environmental, and clinical factors. This approach holds promise for improving treatment outcomes and minimizing side effects.

Genomic Profiling:

Genomic profiling involves analyzing a patient's genetic makeup to spot specific genetic variations related to lupus. This information can help predict disease risk, guide treatment decisions, and identify potential therapeutic targets.

Pharmacogenomics:

Pharmacogenomics studies how genetic variations affect drug response. By understanding how a patient's genetic profile influences their response to medications, healthcare providers can customize drug choices and dosages to optimize treatment.

Precision Medicine Approaches:

Precision medicine approaches use data from genomics, proteomics, and clinical studies to develop individualized treatment plans. This strategy aims to match patients with the foremost effective treatments supporting their unique disease characteristics.

FUTURE DIRECTIONS

Looking ahead, several key areas of research and development hold promise for advancing lupus treatment and improving patient outcomes.

Novel Drug Development:

Continued research into novel drug targets and mechanisms is important for locating new treatment options. Advances in drug discovery technologies and high-throughput screening may cause the event of simpler and targeted therapies.

Improved Disease Monitoring:

Developing more accurate and non-invasive methods for monitoring disease activity and treatment response may be a priority. Advances in imaging technologies, wearable devices, and biosensors may provide valuable tools for real-time disease monitoring.

Integrative and Holistic Approaches:

Integrative and holistic approaches that combine conventional treatments with complementary therapies may offer additional benefits for managing lupus. Research into the efficacy of complementary treatments, like dietary interventions and lifestyle modifications, is ongoing.

Patient-Centered Research:

Engaging patients in research and considering their perspectives in treatment development is crucial. Patient-centered research aims to deal with the requirements and preferences of people with lupus, ensuring that new treatments align with their priorities and improve quality of life.

Global Collaboration:

Global collaboration among researchers, healthcare providers, and patient organizations can accelerate progress in lupus research. International partnerships and data sharing initiatives can enhance our understanding of the disease and drive advancements in treatment.

HOPE AND EMPOWERMENT

As research continues to advance, there's growing hope for improved treatments and a far better understanding of lupus. Staying informed about research developments and participating in clinical trials offers opportunities for accessing new therapies and contributing to the progress of lupus science.

Clinical Trials Participation:

Participating in clinical trials allows individuals with lupus to access cutting-edge treatments and contribute to research. Clinical trials provide valuable data which will cause new treatment options and improved disease management.

Advocacy and Awareness:

Advocating for lupus research and raising awareness about the disease can help drive progress and support funding for research initiatives. Engaging in advocacy efforts and supporting lupus organizations can contribute to positive change within the field.

Patient Empowerment:

Empowering patients with knowledge and resources can enhance their ability to manage lupus and make informed decisions about their care. Education, support, and active participation in treatment planning can improve overall well-being and quality of life.

In the next chapter, we'll explore strategies for managing lupus in specific populations, including children, pregnant women, and older adults. Understanding the unique considerations for these groups can help tailor treatment approaches and support their specific needs.

CHAPTER 9

MANAGING LUPUS IN SPECIFIC POPULATIONS

Lupus affects individuals across various age groups and life stages, each presenting unique challenges and considerations. This chapter explores the management of lupus in specific populations, including children, pregnant women, and older adults, highlighting tailored approaches to treatment and care.

LUPUS IN CHILDREN

Diagnosing and managing lupus in children involves addressing both the disease's impact and therefore the unique developmental needs of younger patients.

Diagnosis:
Pediatric lupus often presents differently from adult lupus. Symptoms may include rash, joint pain, and fever, but also can involve growth delays or more severe organ involvement. Diagnosis in children is often challenging thanks to overlapping symptoms with other conditions, requiring careful evaluation by a pediatric rheumatologist.

Treatment Considerations:

Treatment for pediatric lupus must be carefully managed to balance disease control with growth and development. Pediatric patients often require lower doses of medicines and shut monitoring to avoid potential side effects that would impact growth.

Medications:

Common medications include corticosteroids, immunosuppressants, and hydroxychloroquine. Pediatric doses are adjusted to support weight and age. Long-term use of corticosteroids is monitored closely to attenuate adverse effects on growth and bone health.

Growth and Development:

Regular monitoring of growth and developmental milestones is crucial. Pediatricians and rheumatologists work together to make sure that treatment doesn't negatively impact physical or cognitive development.

Psychosocial Support:

Children with lupus may experience emotional and social challenges thanks to their condition. Support from psychological state professionals, school counselors, and peer support groups can help address issues like anxiety, depression, and social isolation.

School and Social Integration:

Developing a faculty plan that accommodates medical needs is important. This might include managing medication schedules, addressing fatigue, and providing support for missed school days. Collaboration with teachers and faculty staff helps ensure a supportive learning environment.

LUPUS AND PREGNANCY

Pregnancy in individuals with lupus requires careful planning and management to make sure the health of both the mother and therefore the baby.

Preconception Counseling:
Before becoming pregnant, individuals with lupus should consult their healthcare team to assess disease stability and discuss potential risks. This counseling includes reviewing medications, managing disease activity, and planning for a healthy pregnancy.

Disease Control:
Achieving stable lupus disease control before pregnancy is crucial. Uncontrolled lupus can increase the danger of complications like preeclampsia, premature birth, and miscarriage.

Medication Management:
Some lupus medications may have to be adjusted or discontinued during pregnancy. For instance, certain immunosuppressants and corticosteroids can have potential effects on fetal development. Healthcare providers work to seek out the safest medication regimen that balances disease management with fetal health.

Monitoring During Pregnancy:

Regular prenatal visits with a maternal-fetal medicine specialist and a rheumatologist are essential for monitoring the health of both the mother and therefore the baby. Monitoring includes assessing lupus activity, managing potential complications, and ensuring proper fetal growth and development.

Complications:

Potential complications include lupus flares, gestational hypertension, and preterm labor. Close monitoring and timely interventions help manage these risks and ensure a healthier pregnancy outcome.

Postpartum Care:

The postpartum period requires careful monitoring as lupus may reactivate after delivery. Healthcare providers still manage disease activity and adjust medications as required. Postpartum support includes addressing any physical or emotional challenges associated with the recovery and adjustment to parenthood.

LUPUS IN OLDER ADULTS

Managing lupus in older adults involves addressing the intersection of lupus with aging-related health issues.

Diagnosis and Disease Manifestations:

Lupus in older adults may present with atypical symptoms or be confused with other age-related conditions. Older patients may experience different manifestations of lupus, like increased prevalence of joint pain and skin issues. A comprehensive evaluation is important to differentiate lupus from other potential causes.

Treatment Considerations:
Treatment in older adults must consider potential interactions with other medications and existing health conditions, like disorder or osteoporosis.

Medication Management:
Careful selection and dosing of medicines are essential to attenuate side effects and interactions. Corticosteroids and immunosuppressants must be used judiciously, and alternative therapies could also be considered to manage lupus while addressing comorbid conditions.

Chronic Disease Management:
Older adults with lupus often have additional health conditions that need management. Coordinating care among various healthcare providers ensures that each one aspects of health are addressed which treatment plans are integrated.

Bone Health and Osteoporosis:
Long-term use of corticosteroids in older adults can increase the danger of osteoporosis and fractures. Monitoring bone density and implementing preventive measures, like calcium and vitamin D supplementation, are important aspects of care.

Cognitive and Emotional Health:
Lupus and its treatments can impact cognitive and emotional health in older adults. Addressing cognitive changes, like memory issues, and providing psychological state support are important for maintaining overall quality of life.

Support Systems and Resources:

Access to support systems and resources, including community services, caregiver support, and academic materials, can help older adults manage lupus and maintain their independence.

TAILORING LOOK AFTER SPECIAL POPULATIONS

Each population group children, pregnant women, and older adults requires a tailored approach to lupus management. Collaborating with specialists, implementing individualized treatment plans, and addressing the unique needs of every group are key to effective care.

Interdisciplinary Care:
Managing lupus in these specific populations often involves an interdisciplinary approach, including rheumatologists, pediatricians, obstetricians, gerontologists, and other specialists. Coordinated care ensures that each one aspect of health is addressed and treatment plans are comprehensive.

Patient and Family Education:
Providing education to patients and their families about lupus, treatment options, and disease management is crucial. Tailoring education to the precise needs of every population helps improve understanding and adherence to treatment plans.

Advocacy and Support:
Advocacy efforts and support organizations play an important role in addressing the requirements of those populations. Engaging with advocacy groups, accessing resources, and participating in support networks can enhance care and supply valuable assistance.

In the final chapter, we'll discuss the broader impact of lupus on lifestyle and methods for improving overall quality of life. Understanding how lupus affects various aspects of life and exploring strategies for managing these impacts can help individuals lead fulfilling lives despite the challenges of the disease.

CHAPTER 10

LIVING WITH LUPUS: STRATEGIES FOR IMPROVING QUALITY OF LIFE

Lupus may be a chronic condition that affects not only physical health but also emotional well-being, social relationships, and daily functioning. For people with lupus, learning to navigate these challenges and finding ways to enhance their quality of life is important. This chapter explores practical strategies for managing lupus day-to-day, building resilience, and maintaining a satisfying life despite the disease.

MANAGING SYMPTOMS IN DAILY LIFE

One of the first challenges for people with lupus is handling unpredictable and fluctuating symptoms. Effective symptom management requires both proactive strategies and therefore the flexibility to regulate plans as required.

Energy Management and Fatigue:
 Fatigue is one among the foremost common and debilitating symptoms of lupus. Learning to manage energy levels is crucial for maintaining productivity and preventing flare-ups.

Pacing and Prioritization:

Pacing activities and recognizing personal limits help conserve energy. Prioritizing important tasks and delegating or delaying non-essential activities can reduce fatigue and stop overexertion.

Rest and Sleep:

Ensuring adequate rest and a uniform sleep schedule supports the body's healing and recovery processes. Creating a restful environment, practicing good sleep hygiene, and allowing naps during the day can help manage fatigue.

Balanced Exercise:

Although lupus can cause joint pain and fatigue, moderate exercise has been shown to enhance overall health and reduce lupus symptoms. Low-impact activities like walking, swimming, and yoga help maintain mobility, improve mood, and enhance energy levels. However, it's important to balance activity with adequate rest to stop overexertion.

Managing Pain and Joint Stiffness:

Lupus often involves joint pain and stiffness, particularly during flare-ups. Managing this discomfort is important for maintaining mobility and preventing disability.

Physical Therapy:

Working with a physiotherapist can help improve joint function, strengthen muscles, and reduce pain. physiotherapy may include specific exercises, stretching routines, and techniques for managing flare-ups.

Heat and Cold Therapy:

Applying heat to stiff joints can help relax muscles and increase flexibility, while cold packs can reduce swelling and inflammation. Alternating between heat and cold therapy may provide relief during flare-ups.

Medications and Pain Management:

Over-the-counter pain relievers, anti-inflammatory medications, and prescribed drugs can help manage joint pain. Consulting with healthcare providers ensures that pain management strategies are safe and effective.

EMOTIONAL WELL-BEING AND MENTAL HEALTH

The emotional impact of lupus is often profound, and addressing psychological state is as important as managing physical symptoms. Lupus can affect mood, increase stress, and contribute to conditions like anxiety and depression.

Coping with Stress:

Chronic stress can worsen lupus symptoms and trigger flare-ups. Learning to manage stress effectively may be a key part of living with the disease.

Mindfulness and Relaxation Techniques:

Practices like meditation, deep breathing exercises, and progressive muscle relaxation can help reduce stress and promote relaxation. These techniques are particularly helpful during flare-ups or when handling stressors associated with lupus.

Setting Boundaries:

Setting limits with others and learning to mention no can help manage stress and stop overcommitment. Reducing stress in lifestyle by setting boundaries helps preserve energy and stop flare-ups.

Seeking Professional Support:
psychological state professionals, like psychologists or counselors, can provide support for handling the emotional impact of lupus. Cognitive-behavioral therapy (CBT) and other therapeutic approaches can help individuals develop healthy coping strategies, improve mood, and build resilience.

Connecting with Support Networks:
Support from family, friends, and lupus communities plays an important role in emotional well-being. Joining a support group, whether face to face or online, can provide a way of belonging and an area to share experiences with others who understand the challenges of lupus.

SOCIAL LIFE AND RELATIONSHIPS

Lupus can affect social interactions and relationships, as managing the disease often requires lifestyle adjustments and accommodations. Open communication and setting realistic expectations with others are key to maintaining strong relationships.

Communicating with Family and Friends:
Openly discussing lupus with family and friends helps build understanding and support. Explaining the character of lupus, including symptoms like fatigue and pain, can help others adjust their expectations and offer appropriate assistance.

Setting Expectations:

It's important to line realistic expectations with loved ones, especially when it involves participating in social activities. Sharing information about how lupus affects lifestyle and energy levels can prevent misunderstandings and foster empathy.

Asking for Help:

Posing for help when needed is an important part of managing lupus. Whether it's assistance with chores, childcare, or emotional support, counting on a support network can alleviate stress and stop burnout.

Managing Social Activities:

Social activities are often physically and emotionally draining, especially during flare-ups. Balancing social engagements with rest and self-care ensures that individuals with lupus can participate in meaningful activities without exacerbating their symptoms.

Adjusting Plans:

Flexibility is vital when it involves managing social life with lupus. It's important to feel comfortable adjusting or canceling plans if symptoms worsen. Having backup plans and alternative activities can help maintain a social life while respecting personal health needs.

Maintaining Friendships:

Keeping friends involved in one's life, even during times of illness, can strengthen relationships. Simple gestures like texting, calling, or meeting for a brief tea break can maintain connection without overwhelming energy reserves.

WORK AND CAREER CONSIDERATIONS

Lupus can impact business life, but with the proper strategies and accommodations, individuals can successfully manage their careers while living with the disease.

Workplace Accommodations:
Many workplaces offer accommodations for workers with chronic illnesses, like flexible schedules, remote work options, or adjustments to workload. It's important to debate these needs with supervisors and HR departments to make a supportive work environment.

Ergonomic Adjustments:
Adjustments like ergonomic seating, modified workstations, or assistive devices can make the workday easier and reduce physical strain.

Managing Fatigue at Work:
Taking regular breaks, managing workload, and pacing tasks can help prevent burnout during the workday. It's important to prioritize tasks and manage time effectively to balance productivity with health needs.

Career Transitions:
For a few individuals with lupus, their disease may necessitate a career change or modification. Transitioning to a less physically demanding job, or one with more flexible hours, can help maintain a balance between work and health.

DIET AND NUTRITION

Proper nutrition plays a big role in managing lupus symptoms and supporting overall health. While no specific diet can cure lupus, certain foods can help reduce inflammation and promote well-being.

Anti-Inflammatory Foods:

Diets rich in fruits, vegetables, whole grains, and healthy fats can help reduce inflammation and support the system. Omega-3 fatty acids, found in fish like salmon and flaxseeds, are shown to assist manage inflammation.

Avoiding Triggers:

Some individuals with lupus may find that certain foods, like processed foods, refined sugars, and excessive salt, can trigger flare-ups. Keeping a food journal and identifying potential triggers can help manage symptoms.

Hydration:

Staying properly hydrated is important for overall health. Drinking a lot of water throughout the day helps support bodily functions and may alleviate symptoms like joint stiffness and fatigue.

Supplements and Vitamins:

In some cases, healthcare providers may recommend supplements to deal with deficiencies caused by lupus or its treatment. vitamin D and calcium supplements, for instance, can help maintain bone health, especially in individuals taking corticosteroids.

Empowerment and Advocacy

Living with lupus requires resilience, adaptability, and empowerment. Staying informed about the disease, advocating for one's own health, and participating in lupus awareness initiatives can cause greater control over the disease and foster a way of purpose.

Education and Self-Advocacy:

Being an informed patient empowers individuals to form decisions about their care. Learning about lupus, staying up so far with new treatments, and communicating effectively with healthcare providers ensures that patients can advocate for the simplest care.

Participating in Lupus Awareness and Advocacy:

Joining lupus organizations and participating in awareness campaigns can provide a way of community and contribute to positive change. Advocacy efforts help increase research funding, improve access to worry, and lift public awareness of lupus.

Finding Purpose and Fulfillment:

Despite the challenges of lupus, many individuals find new sources of purpose and fulfillment in their lives. Whether through advocacy, creative outlets, or new hobbies, finding activities that bring joy and meaning is important for emotional well-being.

CONCLUSION

Living with lupus presents a variety of challenges, but with the proper strategies and support, it's possible to take care of a top quality of life. Managing this disease requires a multifaceted approach that addresses both the physical and emotional aspects of health. A key element in navigating lupus is learning the way to balance activity and rest, manage stress, and adapt to ever-changing symptoms. While flare-ups can disrupt lifestyle, proactive steps like prioritizing energy management and adopting healthy lifestyle habits can minimize their impact.

Symptom management becomes central to day-to-day living, with careful attention to factors like fatigue, pain, and joint stiffness. Incorporating physiotherapy, practicing mindfulness, and staying active with low-impact exercise are all tools which will enhance well-being. Beyond the physical symptoms, the mental toll of living with lupus can't be overlooked. Individuals have to address the psychological impacts, like anxiety and depression, by seeking professional support and developing coping strategies. Strong support networks be it from family, friends, or lupus communities help alleviate the emotional strain and supply an important buffer during difficult times.

Maintaining social connections and a satisfying business life, though sometimes demanding, is feasible with the proper adjustments. Open communication with loved ones and employers fosters understanding and ensures that accommodations are made when needed. Flexibility in both social and work settings is crucial. As people with lupus learn to adapt to their body's changing needs, they become better at managing their condition while still engaging in activities that bring them joy and purpose.

Diet and nutrition also play a big role in supporting overall health. While there's no definitive lupus diet, it specializes in anti-inflammatory foods and maintaining hydration can help manage symptoms and stop flare-ups. Avoiding known dietary triggers and incorporating the proper supplements under the guidance of a healthcare provider ensures that the body receives adequate nutrition to combat the disease's effects.

Empowerment is probably one among the foremost important elements in living well with lupus. Staying informed about the newest research, treatment options, and self-care techniques allows individuals to require charge of their health. Self-advocacy within the healthcare system, including participation in lupus awareness and advocacy efforts, strengthens the broader community and fosters a way of purpose. Engaging in advocacy not only empowers the individual but also contributes to greater understanding and support for the lupus community at large.

Ultimately, living well with lupus is about finding a balance between rest and activity, between self-care and therefore the support of others, and between accepting the challenges of the disease and still striving for fulfillment. It's about resilience and adaptableness, learning to thrive within the face of uncertainty. With the proper tools and mindset, individuals with lupus can't only manage their condition but also lead meaningful, vibrant lives, proving that lupus could also be a neighborhood of their story, but it doesn't define them.